César Ochoa García

BRAIN, PHYSICAL ACTIVITY AND LEARNING

César Ochoa García

BRAIN, PHYSICAL ACTIVITY AND LEARNING

An indissoluble trinomial

ScienciaScripts

Imprint

Any brand names and product names mentioned in this book are subject to trademark, brand or patent protection and are trademarks or registered trademarks of their respective holders. The use of brand names, product names, common names, trade names, product descriptions etc. even without a particular marking in this work is in no way to be construed to mean that such names may be regarded as unrestricted in respect of trademark and brand protection legislation and could thus be used by anyone.

Cover image: www.ingimage.com

This book is a translation from the original published under ISBN 978-3-639-55555-4.

Publisher:
Sciencia Scripts
is a trademark of
Dodo Books Indian Ocean Ltd. and OmniScriptum S.R.L publishing group

120 High Road, East Finchley, London, N2 9ED, United Kingdom
Str. Armeneasca 28/1, office 1, Chisinau MD-2012, Republic of Moldova, Europe
Printed at: see last page
ISBN: 978-620-6-46743-4

Contents

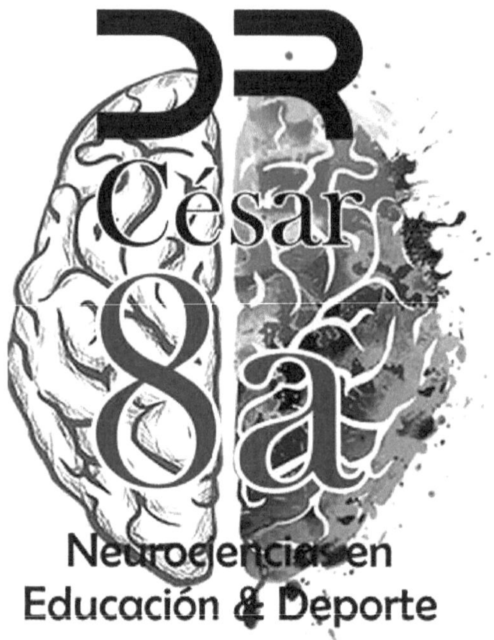

DEDICATION

Son, nothing compares to the joyful happiness of seeing you grow year by year, *you* are the *fruit* of *love and our greatest treasure.*

You have given us a lot of happiness and every day you have given us lessons of teaching and reflection.

You came into my life to be the main driving force in pushing me to be a better person, father and professional.

I want to dedicate this book to you by leaving you the following message for when you are old enough to understand it:

> *"The* easy *part* is done
> *The difficult is done*
> the impossible is attempted".

for you Sebastian

Let's be honest: why is Messi the best player in the world? This or very similar questions are the ones that those of us who work in pants, whether we work in physical education, physical activity for health or sports initiation, ask ourselves on a daily basis. We have not yet found our holy grail, and I have repeatedly stated that it is very likely that we will find in the neurosciences many of the answers we are looking for today.

Fortunately you have in your hands a text that inevitably brings us a little closer to these longed-for answers. It brings us closer to knowledge that seemed far away, it provides us academically and gives us a scientific rigour that we have lost in recent times.

This courageous work, the result of the academic study and school practice of its author - who I have had the pleasure and honour of seeing work and share academic discussions with him - provides us with proposals that will help us to transfer neuroscience to our playgrounds and courts, generating new knowledge.

Read it, discuss it, put it into practice and grow this book.

Daniel Cordoba I lledo
Doctor of Educational Sciences
Barcelona, Catalonia

INTRODUCTION

This book is addressed to all those who are involved in the area of teaching, whether academic or sporting, inviting them to reflect on what we are doing day by day and thus achieve a collective awareness through which we can project our work to society with a higher professional level. In this paper I propose to share reflections, experiences and ideas that have arisen from my own practice as an educator and with this I invite you to meditate on how to make the necessary decisions to achieve significant changes in our respective areas of work. I will try to explain what neuroscience is and what can be achieved with the timely intervention of neuroscience in our teaching sessions. I do not intend to delve into technical concepts that may be diffuse, what I seek is to arouse interest, because I believe that we have in our hands the opportunity to impact on others; therefore, I pose the following question: How can we encourage from our teaching, to a change aimed at being more and better people and a more evolved society?

Currently, in the society in which we live we have challenges that we must address: transforming the teaching-learning process, achieving intellectual autonomy in students, challenging talent and awakening awareness. Many times as teachers we have complained that our work is not recognised, but I ask you, what have you contributed from your area to change the perception of those who criticise you? We can leave the dogmatic arguments and propose with a scientific basis, education in general is nourished by many other sciences that we apply in our classes but do we really know how to explain them and base them from a scientific and pedagogical perspective towards what we intend to achieve in what we teach? The neurosciences today have managed to do this and this is what I will share in the next six chapters.

The neurosciences have allowed us to know how the incorporation of physical exercise, adequate nutrition and a range of life experiences in different environments can form an axis that maintains the health of the individual (emotional, mental, inner and social) as a coadjuvant for learning. We need to expand the frontiers of our work in function of the new knowledge provided by brain science. In recent years, this science has unveiled the mysteries of how the brain works, which has led to important findings for the field of education, since it has provided knowledge to better understand the neural bases of learning, memory, emotions and attention processes that we deal with daily in our teaching work, as well as many other brain functions that are, day by day, stimulated and strengthened in the classroom and in sports institutions.

In the following chapters you will find a set of texts on the relevance of knowing attentional processes to enhance learning, the relationship that the latter has with emotions and memory, as well as important aspects of proper nutrition, all with the sole intention of awakening in you a concern that will generate curiosity to investigate more about this topic that I am passionate about and that I believe that in the coming years will generate changes in the current paradigms of education in the world.

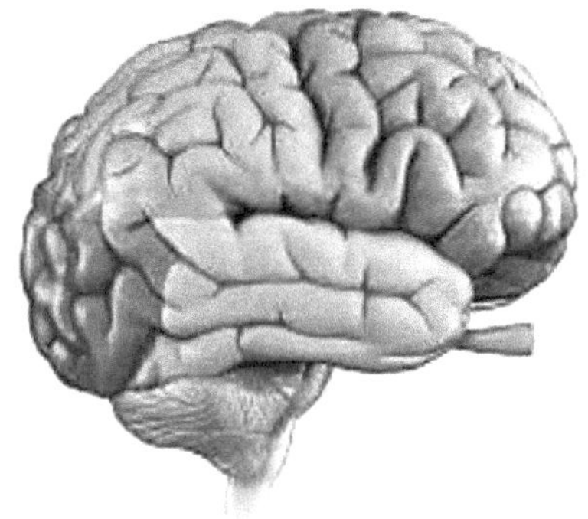

NEUROSCIENCES

Neurosciences: current alternative in education-learning.

Why is it important to know how our brain works for learning? Well, everything is based on the brain, which we could compare to a tree because no two are alike; 500 new facts about the brain are discovered every day (Fisher, 2007), as neuroscience studies are being carried out in many parts of the world. From the studies carried out we can say that the evolution of the brain has taken place in three stages until today:

• Reptilian (middle and small): 500 million years ago; denotes needs such as shelter, toileting and survival.

• L^bic (mammalian brain): 200 million years ago, where emotions and decision-making were prominent.

• Neocortex (rational brain, executive functions present): 10 billion years ago, where rational, language and executive functions are emphasised.

These three brains actually collaborate to make daily decisions in an individual's life, from what to eat today, to what clothes to wear, to what answer to give to a simple question.

The brain is in charge of expressing behaviour, language, thoughts and feelings, but how much do we know about it? Nowadays we no longer talk about the right and left hemispheres as we did years ago. Morgan Priman claimed that we only use 10% of our brain capacity but this has recently been proven to be untrue, we use 2% (quoted in Bachrach, 2015). Nobody can use all they want when they want; you can't turn on all the neurons even if you want to, because they have a limited capacity for ene^a. The brain is electricity, physical and chemical, you can only turn on 2% of the wiring inside you at the same time, otherwise you would melt it down. eWe use all our neurons? SG at the same time? No, but we have billions of possible connections.

On the other hand, there is the mind, which is made up of thoughts and emotions. The mind is what happens to the brain; analogously speaking, you build it every day, because it depends on what you think. In sport, for example, you practice a physical skill and if you repeat it constantly, you become mechanised and automated; in basketball, you could make a shot at the basket even without seeing, but if you don't adjust your neural wiring by trying new things you'll just be good at shooting at the basket. So when you are faced with a game situation where you have to make decisions in a matter of seconds, you might not be able to make a smart play but mechanised.

The training we have received for centuries has not been oriented towards the functioning of our body-brain-mind unit (BCMU). Recent research indicates that stress and emotional disorders are on the rise and people are unable to master their emotional states. It is important to achieve the ability to regulate impulses, increase empathy, manage interpersonal relationships, as well as develop and preserve reasoning faculties; for this science shows that learning is the key to human progress. We must achieve a knowledge-oriented education, so that it becomes an effective method of individual growth, conflict resolution and development of values, which are essential factors in achieving personal and group success and happiness.

Neuroscience in education today

The knowledge of neuroscience is transforming both the content and the perspective of classic problems according to Mora (2017): what is the cerebral basis of the mental? can the emotional and the cognitive be differentiated? Today, among the educational community and anyone interested in the phenomenon of learning, there is a need to learn about a new discipline derived from neuroscience: neuroeducation.

Neuroeducation or neurodidactics is a bridging discipline between neurology and educational science. It is a renewed vision of teaching, based on the brain, which takes advantage of the knowledge of scientific research on how the brain works. It integrates psychology, sociology and medicine; it seeks to enhance the processes of learning and memory, taking advantage of the latest scientific knowledge on emotion, attention and memory; it puts the triad of family, social environment and culture into perspective and explains how they influence the success or failure of the individual. These are determinants of learning ability, recognising their variability, both in genetics and in the changes that the environment produces in the brain.

Neuroeducation helps to detect psychological or brain processes that may interfere with learning and memory, as well as with education itself. Recent studies recommend applying in the classroom knowledge about the brain processes of emotion, curiosity and attention; that is to say, methods adapted to joy and to awaken pleasure in the learning activity itself, to enjoy learning, something that we often forget because we are immersed in the world of technology. This technology that has been evolving to make our daily tasks easier, many times we use it wrongly, for example, a mobile phone nowadays allows us to keep many contacts and I assure you that if at this moment I ask you to tell me five contact numbers of your friends or relatives with whom you communicate the most, surely you will not be able to remember the five numbers; when this electronic device did not exist we easily remembered telephone numbers because we practised and used our memory, nowadays we no longer exercise it, as the mobile phone stores them and we only have to touch a few keys to obtain them. We no longer exercise our memory and memory is essential for the complex process of learning to take place correctly.

The following is a representative graph of the above mentioned

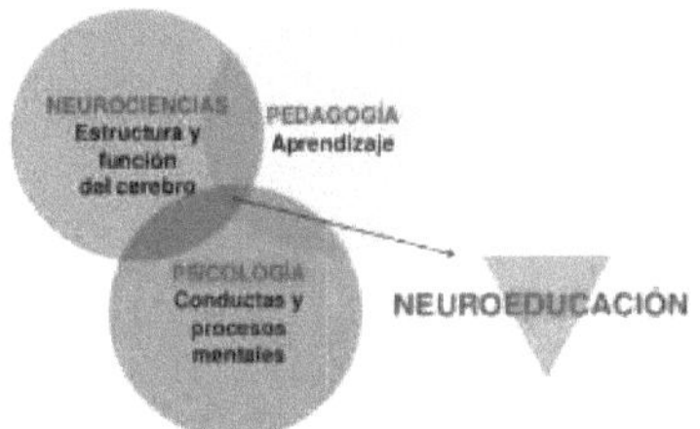

Source: blogs.larepublica.pe

In our days, it is notorious that the interest of the students is being lost more and more, they are no longer interested in learning, they do not find the sense nor the motivation to do it and they do not want to go to school to learn more every day. If the teacher knew that the synaptic changes that occur in the brain are the result of the teaching that the students receive, he/she would surely transform his/her attitude, favouring a different tone, both emotionally and cognitively, at the time of teaching. In addition to this, we have to consider that brain development occurs asynchronously, it has different times, which we could describe as windows that open at a certain time, when certain information from the environment (sensory, motor, family, social, emotional) enters them, and no other time - period of myelination - is more optimal than that.

Therefore, neurosciences have positioned themselves in the educational field, generating psychoneuroeducation, which is an educational system developed by Dr. Carlos Logatt Grabner as a result of the integration of the most recent neuroscientific advances and other related disciplines that focus on the knowledge, understanding and modelling of behaviour or, in other words, respect for oneself and others and the development and growth as human beings (Logatt, 2013).

On the other hand, there is neuroeducation, which is an interdiscipline that promotes a greater integration between the sciences of education and those that deal with the neuroscientific development related to learning and teaching in all its forms, generating a new profession, as neuroscience in sport has recently begun to be talked about, a subject that has gained a lot of strength.

In summary, the neurosciences in the teaching-learning framework study how the brain interacts with its environment in relation to learning, the chemical, pharmacological and pathological structure and function of the nervous system and how the different elements of the nervous system interact and give rise to behaviour.

Methodology on which neurosciences are based

Neuropsychoeducation focuses its work on information and memory. It seeks to educate in order to keep the higher cognitive faculties of the brain active, which allow emotional and instinctive responses to be made conscious, developing:

- The   ability to understand
- The   analyticalcapacity
- The   evaluation   capacity

The methodology is based on two premises:

a)   Transforming the complex statements of science into a more easily understandable language, accessible to all.

b)   Select, analyse, evaluate and organise the large amount of scattered scientific material.

Underpinning disciplines

In the text "Neuroeducation for all" Logatt mentions the following disciplines:

- Behavioural genetics
- Behavioural sociology
- Evolutionary psychology
- Genetics
- Memetica
- Evolution
- Preventive medicine
- Nutrition
- Sociology

Neuroscience in sport

There has long been a myth, as I mentioned earlier, that we have a right and a left hemisphere that work separately, but this is not so^ they work at the same time. If we had the opportunity to visualize our brain through a nuclear magnetic resonance, we could observe how different areas of both hemispheres light up at the same time, some more than others according to the activity of each side. The brain is electricity (physical and chemical) and we use it all, although we cannot use all the neurons at the same time, as it is only possible to switch on simultaneously 2% of our neurons, which is equivalent to 31 million possible connections.

The greater the learning, the greater the number of neuronal connections, which is equivalent to more intelligence. In sports, we say to the athlete that he has to believe in his capacity and motor performance in the sport he plays; in the case of football, the technical part does not depend on the foot, but on the brain, which allows the process by which the foot kicks the ball, to which is added the sporting talent. If the player learns more new things about his sport, he will be a more intelligent player, with more neural connections. In other words, in sport 90% is in the mind and 10% in the head, i.e. in the brain. The mind is a term that sometimes we do not understand and it is necessary to clarify that this is not the brain, it is different; the brain is matter and the mind is thought and emotions.

For those involved in sport Bachrach (2015) said that there are four key elements to work on in order to reach the maximum potential and maintain it at an optimal level:

1. Mental ability: achieving cognitive flexibility in decision-making.
2. Regulating emotions: Intensify them or reduce their intensity.
3. Visualisations: Imagining that you have already achieved your planned goal.
4. Intrinsic motivation: to do it simply for the pleasure and enjoyment it brings.

To get better at what we do, be it school or sport, then we must consider the creation of new neural circuits as synonymous with learning. In sport, if you learn new moves and strategies, you will be considered a smarter player; this will also depend on the motivation of the player and whether the player has the right environment, because if the player is under too much stress, this will translate into stress and in turn into less learning.

If you are interested in knowing the most recent discoveries in relation to sport it is necessary to mention that the most important sports centres in the world are:

- Howard Hughes Medical Institute, North Western University Consid USA.
- University of Ulister, Ireland.
- Department of Physical Education, State University of Birmingham.
- Departament Staps Faculte des Sciences de L'homme et de Lenviroment, Universite de la Reunion, France.

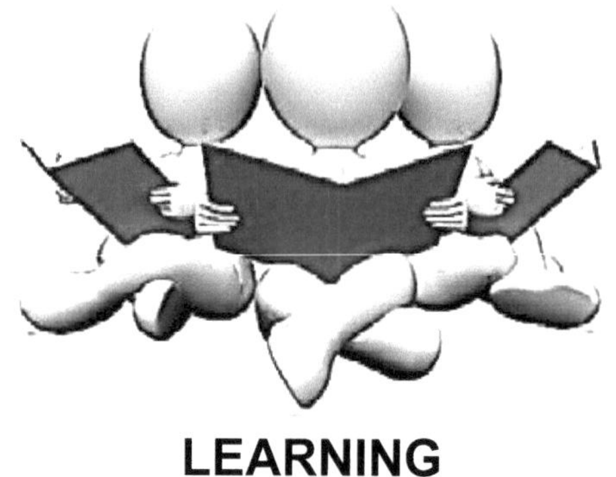

LEARNING

LEARNING: BEYOND KNOWLEDGE

Today we have the desire to learn and to know something that is useful for society; for this we must develop an individual with the specific aptitudes to learn in the new social scenarios. For this, it is necessary to know how the stimuli of modernity operate in our brain structures and the basic physiology of learning, in order to correlate them with behaviours and habits.

Neurosciences explain the term learning as the process by which experiences modify our nervous system and from there our behaviour. To become learning specialists we have to know how to prioritise stimuli, as well as how to re-elaborate the interpretations of reality in order to modify its subjectivity, as intelligence is a modifiable concept. An expert incorporates healthy eating habits and physical exercise because he knows their impact on learning. Good rest contributes to produce metaconscious associations for creativity, for the conceptual linkage between neural modules and for the consolidation of what has been learned; behaviour is produced by the neural networks that have been able to link.

Let us now focus a little on the learning process, the factors involved in it and how we have omitted situations that could favour it for school, sport, social situations and personal goals, to name a few. Learning and memorising change synaptic wiring, activities we perform from birth to death. Learning is one of the most complex functions of the human brain and involves an adequate level of mental alertness and concentration. Learning is the first brain mechanism required to become aware of something, and it is worth noting that the brain and exercise are allies in learning.

Rosler (2014) mentions that the movement has six purposes:

1. Preparing the brain
2. Providing brain breaks
3. Stimulating health and exercise
4. Developing cohesion in the classroom
5. Reviewing the content
6. Teaching the content

Learning takes a moment of effort until it becomes conscious, automatic. At the beginning the handling of so much information tires you, but when you practice more, you automate it and it becomes easier, for example driving a car. Learning, for a child in a context full of sounds, colours and shapes, is simply pleasurable and intense. Play is an emotional mechanism by which the child acquires skills and abilities through the whirlwind of changes that his brain makes at high speed.

Spedonic physical movement prepares the brain for learning by providing a pleasant and welcoming learning environment. These specific exercises improve neural connections; as neurons communicate, cognitive abilities are enhanced. When we exercise both hemispheres, concentration is improved through hemispheric dissociation exercises, examples of which are given at the end of the book.

At school one must learn to plan, organise and classify the knowledge acquired in cooperation with others; to learn, memorise and relate to others is to acquire abilities and skills that will serve inside and outside the school, so learning is to acquire fluency of thoughts and emotions that lead to making a social decision lead us to control our behaviours and actions, to have control over what we think, say and do.

If you were to turn to the infographic on learning: what percentage do we learn with each sense by Piktochartz, you would find the following: hearing 11%, smell 3.5%, touch 1.5%, taste 1% and sight 83%.

Vestibular system

You need to know a little about the vestibular system, which is the one that gives information to the brain related to monitoring movement (head and body position in space); it is also connected to academic skills, as it is crucial for cognitive functioning. Spatial recognition allows us to recognise objects around us in space and the position of our body in space, without this there will be difficulties in:

- Literacy
- Organisation of written work
- Understanding mathematical concepts
- Reproduction of mathematical concepts and forms

How can I help to improve the vestibular system and thus spatial perception? This is very simple: with rotational movements, balancing movements, jumps and turns. If you use more of your senses to learn, the perceived and processed information goes into long-term memory and is easier to remember.

Brain breaks

Have you ever found that when you're in a class getting a lot of information, you start to feel distant, diffuse and your attention starts to wander? Studies have shown that it is necessary to provide brain breaks, that is, to give the brain a rest so that it can process information better. One thing that strikes me about schools is that the teacher worries about finishing the subjects, but are the students learning all the subjects or are they just being taught? Also, when we sit for too long, 90% of the brain's oxygen stagnates; we need to take deep breaths or get up and move around, because too little oxygen equals concentration and memory problems.

Rodriguez (2016) discusses what happens when we use brain breaks. The advantages of providing brain breaks are:

- You give the hippocampus (gateway to memory) time to process the information.
- You reduce the feeling of being overwhelmed.
- You bring in the laughter and fun
- You refresh the nervous system
- Brain-body reorganisation

Allowing movement in the classroom or performing specific activities that involve the elements of attention, memory and emotion on the courts will help to enhance learning; getting up and doing quick exercises allows the brain to refocus and gives oxygen to the nervous system. The benefits are:

- Energising the body
- Improve   it   health
- Improve   the   performance   performance
- Improve   the   status   condition
- Improve   the   state   emotional state
- Learn effectively
- Reduce stress

Is it possible for movement to have such an effect on learning, think about the last time you sat for a long time to learn something new - what was your emotional state like? Through movement, learning can be made fun, interesting and exciting. If information is connected to movement, retaining and remembering is easier. When we learn through movement we absorb more information and remember more, it is for all ages, it builds bridges between body and brain. Compare your emotional state when you learned something theoretical just by listening to when you did it by moving, for example skating, swimming and driving a car, think about the learning process. Using your body to incorporate the concept of driving helped you understand it. If someone had given you a theoretical lesson without the practical part to teach you this, would you have achieved this skill?

Examples:

- Understand the concept of a comma in grammar: students walk around saying a sentence and stop every time there is a comma to represent its purpose, thus internalising this.

- Understanding war: students role-play a war situation from history.

Understanding an atom: pupils form it with their bodies.

Movement should not modify the way it is taught, but complement it. It has the following benefits:

- Increasing retention and comprehension
- Improving social skills and group cohesion
- Increasing motivation

How physical activity helps improve learning

The brain learns, as I mentioned earlier, by processing sensory information from the environment, forming networks of neurons through chemical connections (synapses) that help consolidate data. Without a sense of interest or emotional connection to the content, it is easily forgotten; for information to pass from working memory to the associative cortex (long-term memory), which is the holy grail and the goal of learning, something must happen to the information or experience.

There are five ways in which the brain deposits information in long-term memory:

- Semantic: the meaning of words using speech and reading.
- Episodic: this is spatial memory when it creates images of where you were when an event occurred.
- Emotional: processes emotionally charged events.
- Automatic: information that is already automatic with use.
- Motor: information related to movement.

On the other hand, the cerebellum is responsible for the coordination of movement, for example:

- Balance
- Cognitive functions
- Memory

The brain pays attention to the movement, if it is done with a purpose, it keeps the attention and focuses the student. Here are some other benefits of this brain-physical activity pairing:

- Learning is easier to remember, deposit and retrieve if it has an emotional component.
- Gives time to process academic content
- Stimulates health and exercise, refocuses attention
- The brain naturally learns to be stimulated by emotion and movement.
- Movement in the form of prolonged aerobic exercise increases cognitive function and memory, improves attention and stimulates neurons to connect with each other to form new synapses, which is the neurobiological basis of learning.

The nervous system learns through sensory cues, i.e. the more senses you use, the easier it is to learn information. Sitting for too long will cause blood to accumulate in the lower limbs, causing less cerebral blood flow and in turn generating an undesirable learning state. On the other hand, if you allow yourself some time to move, you will alleviate this reduction in blood flow, because when you increase the frequency and strength of muscle contraction, more oxygen reaches your brain.

Recent scientific studies help to justify motor action in cognitive development. Such is the case of Ratey (2008), who explains how exercise activates the brain, specifically the prefrontal cortex, which is responsible for functions such as: organising, initiating or postponing responses, planning, evaluating, learning from errors and maintaining attention. In turn, Monti (2012) and Chaddock (2010) argue that exercise significantly improves relational memory, which allows us to link memories of our experiences. Also, Wendy Suzuky (2011) has argued in her research that exercise, in addition to improving learning and memory, has a positive effect on creativity and imagination.

Here are some of the positive effects that physical activity, if well systematised, has on our organism:

- Provides neuroprotective capacity, counteracting the effects of ageing.

- It helps to generate more neurons.
- Improves executive functions, performance of complex tasks and problem solving.
- It fires the prefrontal cortex, which is responsible for planning, organising, initiating or postponing responses, and maintaining attention, among other functions.
- It pumps up brain chemicals such as BDNF, which is like a biological link between thought, emotion and movement, which increases learning by developing attention-motivation-memory, preparing neurons to grow and expand. It also offers options in the growth and repair of the N.C.S., reversing the loss of the hippocampus. In addition, it achieves the benefits that ritalin, prozac and morphine give to our organism.
- Increases brain mass, enhancing cognitive processing.
- Increases oxygen consumption and hippocampal volume.
- Intense physical activity helps to consolidate learning better and improves long-term memory, because it stimulates the secretion of substances such as noradrenaline and BDNF.
- It improves relational memory, the memory that allows us to link memories to generate our knowledge of the world from our personal experiences.
- Increased blood flow, resulting in increased brain activity.
- Many of these benefits are due to the increased ability of the blood cells to absorb oxygen, improving lung, muscle, heart and brain function.
- Improves the ability to concentrate.
- Generates new blood vessels in the brain (angiogenesis) for learning and health.
- Apart from improving learning and memory, it has effects on creativity and imagination.
- Increases cognitive flexibility, i.e. the ability to pay attention to several tasks at the same time or to switch from one task to another quickly.
- It helps to maintain the grey matter, responsible for data transmission and agility of thought; some diseases and age diminish and destroy it.
- It slows down brain ageing by reversing the ageing of the hippocampus.

Sound and brains

After a good session of physical activity, it is important to get a good night's rest, because only if you sleep well will melatonin appear. This hormone, released at night, is a powerful antioxidant that supports fundamental systems in our organism: the immune, hormonal and cerebral systems.

Sleep is a determining factor in brain neuroplasticity, which is the ability of the nervous system to change its structure and function throughout life, as a reaction   to the diversity of the environment.

environment. It maintains certain synapses and eliminates others, reinforces connections between cortical areas, as well as cognitive processes, mainly the consolidation of memory. It also enhances learning and reinforces those areas related to motor learning. Its absence produces stress, so care must be taken, because when it becomes chronically stressed, glucorticoids are released, which damage the synapses between neurons, particularly the hippocampus, altering the execution of plans and the coordination of movements.

Motor skills as aids to learning

When we are involved in the educational and sporting system, we are familiar with educational currents, theories and various authors who focus on the teaching-learning process (developmental theories, for example); however, we do not stop to consider what some physical qualities determine or whether these were correctly stimulated at the right time. Here are some of them:

Tone: responsible for attention, alertness and activation of mental states. It reflects the first degree of neurological maturation.

Balance: without proper postural control, the brain does not learn.

Laterality: if there is a correct laterality, there will be an optimal maturation, generating improvements in the capacity of perception, analysis and storage of information.

Bodily notion: its absence is tantamount to learning problems and personality disturbances.

Space-time structuring: causes visual and auditory perception problems if not correctly developed.

Our learning is sustained by biological changes in neuronal connections, that is to say, the acquisition of knowledge, even if it is of a sporting nature, generates that qwmical and morphological modifications are provoked in the brain structures.

Our brain has the capacity to modify its own neurochemistry.

Neurons in action

Research in the area of cognitive and social neuroscience has found that emotional and social skills such as self-awareness, self-awareness, self-regulation or autonomy and resilience are usually more important than IQ for both academic and athletic success.

We have heard and heard all the time about neurons. There are myths about them, such as whether they die and do not regenerate again - although in the year 2000 it was detected and confirmed that neurogenesis exists, which is the birth of new neurons in the human brain throughout life - or the effects of drugs on them. I will tell you a little about them: the neuron is the elementary unit of information processing and transmission in the nervous system and acts as a receiver of information coming from other neurons. This information is passed from one neuron to another, transmitted via the synapse, which consists of the junction of a terminal button (presynaptic neuron) with a dendritic spine or with the surface of the cell body (postsynaptic neuron). When neurons are stimulated, a rapid reversal of the membrane potential occurs, which is called an action potential. This produces an electrical current along the axon and the release of neurotransmitters which diffuse through the synaptic space.

The learner interprets new knowledge while linking it to previously formed neural networks; he compares, relates, connects, understands and links, giving rise to a new memory. Therefore, we can say that learning consists of interneuronal synaptic development in networks, which constitute the physical support of the register of experience. The experiences we have change the neural networks and cause changes in behaviour; this is the principle of the term known as neural plasticity. This is the physical change in our brains as a result of experience and learning, leading to new interpretations of the world in which we live. On the other hand, there is the plasticity of the nervous system: the ability of nerve cells to modify the intensity of synapses.

The main function of learning is survival, as survival depends on the knowledge and control we have of the outside world. Thus, learning can be described as the incorporation of new capacities to the demands of the surrounding environment. In other words, learning is the formation and modification of neural networks that make sense of the individual's inner world.

Mirror neurons

In 2010, Roy Murkamel of the University of California first provided information on the existence of mirror neurons in humans. Many of these cells were detected in the hippocampus and in the premotor cortex (the one that deals with learning sequential acts); these neuronal nuclei are activated when we see other people perform an intentional action, for example, if we see someone take a fruit to eat, our mirror neurons will be activated and try to imitate the action. We can say that they are a group of cells that were discovered by the team of neurobiologist Giacomo Rizzolatti and related to the empathic, social and imitative behaviours and their mission is to reflect the activity that we are observing another individual doing. Recall that neurons are the structural and functional unit in our nervous system, the parts that compose them are: the soma or cell body, the dendrites and the axon. The soma or perikaryon or cell body is the main part of the neuron and its function is to allow nerve impulses to travel faster.

Experts assume that they play an important role in cognitive abilities related to social life, such as empathy - the ability to put oneself in the place of another - and imitation - fundamental to learning processes - the mirror neuron is one of the discoveries of the last decade.

One of their characteristics is that they not only allow you to reflect what you are looking at outside yourself on a motor level, but also on an emotional level, as they are connected to the Kmbic system - related to the regulation of emotions, memory and attention-. There are studies that show that children who imitate and observe the facial expressions of others, show a greater activation of these neurons, and the greater the activation, the greater the empathy they show. For example, if a child sees someone smiling, their mirror neurons create an internal simulation of that smile in their brain, send these signals to the hmbic system and end up feeling the same as the person smiling. Therefore, when you are in the period of learning behaviours and emotional responses, it becomes necessary to observe and imitate the reactions of those around you, which end up establishing your own experience. Therefore, whether in sports or in learning another sport, imitation is indispensable.

Recent studies by Gregory Hickock of the University of California (2013) indicated that the mirror neuron system is limited to action comprehension and mimicry that is associated with the perception of movement. Such neurons have opened up a new understanding of how humans connect with each other. Neuroscientist Christian Keysers says: "if you want to connect and collaborate with someone, you have to know what emotional state they are in" (2016).

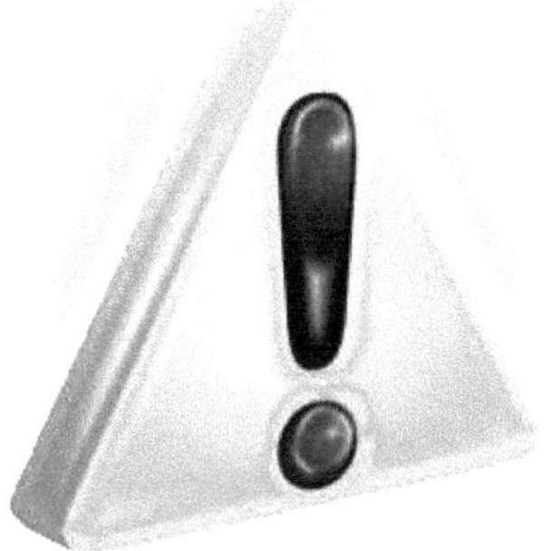

ATTENTION

ATTENTION: KEY TO BETTER PERFORMANCE

Concentration or attention

We can define attention as the ability to understand things, it is a quality of perception that functions as a filter of environmental stimuli, deciding and prioritising through concentration, as well as enabling a better understanding of ourselves and our environment. It also controls and regulates cognitive processes, from learning by conditioning to complex reasoning. In other words, it is the selective application of consciousness to an object or situation. It has three elements:

a) Cognitive: in charge of processing the information you receive. It is when you accommodate the ideas that you already have with the recent information.

b) Emotional: is when you trigger a reaction.

The psychophysiological changes in your body due to perceived information and stimuli, to which you will react positively or negatively.

c) Motor: is when you perform a behavioural action related to what you have learned or information you have received.

When you manage to control and develop these three elements, you determine your slow or fast learning, as you will be solely responsible for initiating, maintaining or stopping attention.

I will explain the above with an example: imagine that you meet an important person, whom you admire and from whom you want to learn something new. This person is an expert, and someone tells you that he is very demanding, does not like to be interrupted and does not allow opinions of what he is saying; cognitively you will get an idea of his personality, maybe you will experience a certain not so nice feeling towards this character, predisposing you before interacting. As you get to know him/her, you will eventually express negative behaviour when facing him/her. But imagine that this behaviour would be different if you had been told the opposite: that he is very open, nice and likes to joke around, making the moment fun for you when he is teaching you something. All the processing would be the opposite of the above.

On the other hand, the rapid processing of information and decision making depend on the nervous system, here concentration plays an important role, for example, a player must always be concentrated on the game and not focused on the play; there are players who tire quickly by the degree of focus on a play, to concentrate is to fix your thoughts and/or attention on something without being distracted, it is a form of selective attention that allows you to process the information that really interests you. The correct concept for this is "focus of attention", according to Reyes (2018) is to focus all the senses on the task we are executing. Athletes who have made it to the top have done so because they have managed to direct their attention to a specific task by completely eliminating any external distractions around them.

Memory goes hand in hand with attention and stores cognitive, emotional and motor elements, and is regulated by neurological centres that must function properly. Any functional or organic alteration will affect its processes and results.

Attention is the brain mechanism required to be aware of something. The mechanism of attention links neurons scattered in the cerebral cortex and thalamus, activating the mechanism of consciousness. With attention, as with perceptions, one learns and memorises. It follows curiosity. There are four types of attention:

- Focused: when you read a book.
- Sustained: when you take a class.
- Selective: when you maintain it in the face of distractions.
- Directive: when you decide and control where to focus it.

They pay attention to cognitive, emotional and motor elements.

Mindfulness

Mindfulness is the exercise in which the mind is fixed on an object and remains attentive to it without any judgement or goal, returning attention to the object after any distraction. It is also considered as mindfulness, an ability to maintain attention in the present in a deliberate way, following the indications of Collard (2014).

We could also say that it is a mental training, an addition that is not superfluous in daily training in sport. When concentration is lost and stress sets in, your nerves contract and your muscles contract, making you less efficient. In addition, your heart rate speeds up, causing a decrease in your ability to make good decisions. This is when your performance is at its worst and you are at the greatest risk of injury.

Meditative activity has been found to promote sensory integration, harmonisation and attunement or synchronisation of the various neural areas, circuits and processes involved in a mental experience. Studies have shown how meditation is associated with structural changes in areas of the brain important for sensory, cognitive and emotional processing. If the brain meditates, it displays a plurality of faculties related to self-control, attention, concentration, impulse control, self-awareness, and so on. If you wanted to teach a child ways of self-control to reduce his impulsivity and aggressiveness, you would have to focus on activities to improve attention.

Fitness-brain relationship

One of the main arguments that explains how motor action contributes to learning and cognitive development according to de Sousa (2014) is that animals have brains and plants do not; the former can move at will and the latter cannot. In this sense you can find in the scientific literature an endless number of benefits that exercise produces in the brain, such is the example of neurologist Fernando Gomez Pinilla of UCLA University, who claims that the brain we have was formed through exercise. His hypothesis states that our genes require exercise and failure to do so may be a factor in new brain diseases such as depression, bipolar disorder, Alzheimer's, among others. Supporting this view, the findings of Marc Roig (2012) show that intense physical activity helps to better consolidate learning and long-term memory; other studies have shown that exercise stimulates the secretion of some memory-enhancing substances such as norepinephrine or BDNF (brain-derived neurotrophic factor).

In the last five years there has been a lot of research on physical activity and its relationship to changes in different areas of the brain. Some studies have shown alterations in the hippocampus (responsible for memory and emotional processes) and others in the prefrontal cortex. Other research in laboratories shows that aerobic physical exercise improves BDNF, a protein responsible for the growth of new neurons and the synapses between them, and its importance in long term memory is recognised. The term neurotrophic refers to any biological factor that participates in the correct formation of neuronal networks in the brain, establishing solid synapses.

Common conditions and their effects on learning

Below I will briefly describe some of the most common conditions, which go unnoticed due to a lack of knowledge of what they can cause in our organism. These alter or affect important functions for our effective performance in academic tasks, sports or simply for our life in general.

TOBACCO: in newborns causes poor response to sensory stimuli.

ANXIETY: diminishes the process of attention, learning and memory, cortical neuronal mechanisms generating impulsivity.

STRESS: causes low attention.

BAD SLEEP: affects the speed of information processing and memory. Signs such as apathy, listlessness, irritability are derived from insufficient sleep.

LOW OXYGEN: affects concentration and memory.

NEGATIVE EMOTIONS: cause a malfunction of the prefrontal cortex.

DEHYDRATION: affects learning, concentration and memory as it damages the frontal lobe responsible for intellectual functions, planning and attention control.

MENTAL AGOBIOUSNESS: lack of sleep, irritability and inattention. It affects brain structures such as the hippocampus, learning processes, memory and emotional development.

The value of proper sensory integration

In the 1960s, Jean Ayres discovered that there are learning problems due to atypical sensory processing. Sensory integration is an unconscious process of the brain, it organises the information detected by the senses and gives meaning to experiences. It also enables us to act and is the basis of learning. The prefrontal cortex plays an important role in coordinating our activities, talents and creative abilities; it allows us to achieve the maximum level of coordination between thinking and feeling. Adequate sensory integration begins in the womb, as it is known that the foetus feels the movements.

If we talk about sensory integration, it is necessary to talk about the importance of crawling, something that many people overlook during a child's development. Crawling is a medial hemispheric reflex, i.e. it affects both sides of the hemisphere, because the involvement of coordinated hand and foot movements stimulates hemispheric integration. If this exchange of sensory information is not stimulated, interhemispheric communication becomes more difficult; when crawling, cross movements are made and the neural connections of the corpus callosum are stimulated. If you are a coach, you should know this in order to understand the reasons for the poor motor responses of your athletes, this will allow you to reorient your tasks to support them so that they can overcome these brakes in their sporting evolution.

Contributions of neuroscience to sport

Before, athletes and coaches focused on the acquisition of motor patterns, on strengthening the muscular bone and cardiorespiratory system, among others, that is to say, the paradigm was centred on the body. Today it is known that there are other factors that were not considered before and that occur at the cerebral level, such as psychological-mental preparation. It is necessary to know what happens in the brain when we acquire a sporting gesture, how sporting performance affects emotional states such as happiness or depression and to understand the incidence of different factors in motor learning, factors which are mentioned below:

- Fatigue
- Thirst
- Fear
- Anxiety
- I sound
- Hunger
- Alegria
- Sadness

The brain is the one that provides all the motor possibilities, it is essential for memorising the sporting technique, whatever it may be, and it provides the emotional modulation that will allow the athlete to obtain his or her maximum level of performance. All this leads us to think of a didactic revolution of learning in the field of training and sport.

The practice of sport involves important brain areas, such as the frontal lobes; but more importantly, it is the cerebellum that ensures the mechanisation of the complex sequences of the specific movements of each sport, as it sends signals to millions of cells in the body, ordering the actions we need to execute. The more practice there is, the easier it will be to remember which nerve circuits and muscle fibres are necessary for a given task.

Another factor to note is the am^gdala, this is a small structure of the Kmbic system that regulates our emotional reactions. Its activation or inhibition will allow us to achieve a better performance at key moments. When the athlete receives boos, cheers, etc., he maximises his state of alertness; he must control the limits of the field of play that correspond to him depending on his position, the ball in movement, the proximity and intentions of the opponent. All this activates the am^gdala.

Finally, the frontal lobes control the reaction of the am^gdala by modulating its emotional arousal. eHow do we achieve this? It is very simple, by controlling breathing and relaxing the muscles, which lowers the heart rate. If you are afraid or too euphoric you provoke an over activation of the Kmbic system, generating interferences in the concentration and in the coordination of your sport gestures.

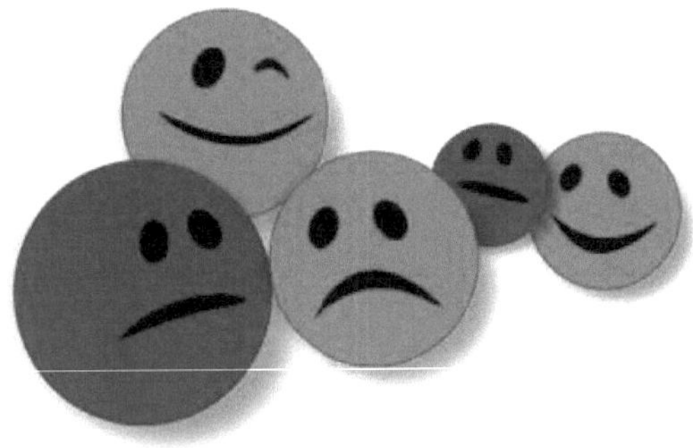

CHAPTER 4

EMOTIONS

EMOTIONS: SUBSTANTIAL TO SUCCESS OR FAILURE

Emotions are something we do not take into account when teaching and have been found to be an important factor in learning. We could define them as ene^a coded in certain circuits of the brain, without them we would be depressed and listless. It activates and maintains curiosity and attention, i.e. emotions awaken the interest in discovering something new, they also serve to evoke memories effectively and are biochemical elements to which the body reacts and activates associative networks in the memory, either negatively or positively. When you experience an emotion, a window opens in your brain, through which you learn and memorise information about the world around you, and this is totally dependent on the type of experience you are facing.

In the vast majority of schools, children are taught cognitively complex concepts in an aseptic way, devoid of emotional meaning. The teacher must take into account that emotions are unconscious mechanisms and feelings, on the contrary, are the conscious experience of a certain emotion. Feelings lead us to know emotions, fear, pleasure and frustration. Emotions are always felt in the body, they are impulses to act, to alter attention and to activate associative networks in the memory. When we teach and want learning to be effective, it is important to consider them. To teach is to move learners, to touch their hearts and minds through their bodies.

What does it mean to regulate emotions?

When we talk about regulating emotions, impulses or desires, we basically want to intentionally reduce or increase the intensity of an emotion and decide whether to proceed following an impulse or desire. This is applicable in sport situations to achieve what we planned before the match; even when we are going to do an exam or an oral presentation if we are motivated by the result, it will change the way we process the information to be learned and it will be easier to study or learn a game strategy, to mention an example.

This emotion regulation includes skills such as:

- Decide and control where to focus attention.
- Deciding and controlling when and how much attention one wants to pay to different aspects of the situation, including one's own thoughts, feelings and impulses.
- Stop yourself from following a sudden impulse.
- Thinking, imagining and doing things that soothe when you feel angry, anxious, afraid, etc.

If we talk about emotions we cannot overlook perception, the five senses tell us what is going on, through them we perceive reality. Each individual perceives reality differently according to their moods and experiences. For example: imagine that one day you leave your house to go to work and you are waiting for the bus and it takes a long time to pass, usually in this situation you start to get annoyed, the delay in passing causes you to be late and your boss looks at you badly when he notices this, then you start to get angry, then when you go to eat near your work they serve you the food poorly, then from annoyance and anger you pass to anger, turning this into a negative spiral. Instead, you can take this in a different way, if the bus doesn't run, you will inevitably be late, but you can use this time to check your diary or check emails on your mobile phone, etc. When you arrive at work and realise that your boss is looking at you in annoyance, you can ignore it because you know it wasn't really your fault and you will get on with your work without it affecting your efficiency, and if they served you the fna meal instead of exploding at the waitress you can ask why they served it like that^ -there will probably be an explanation and you will be compensated for it- instead of having negative emotions. One thing to know about this is that the more negative thoughts you have, the more the right frontal cortex is activated, generating situations such as envy, hostility and frustration, i.e. self-generated unhappiness.

The prefrontal cortex uses thinking and problem-solving strategies. When it doesn't work it is because a negative emotional state is present. 98% of our decisions are emotional, to do something is because our emotional networks within us are being activated. Do you know the emotional state of your students or athletes? Can you manage it?

Elements to improve emotional state:

- Humour
- Music
- Movement

How you do in your life, be it work, school or a sporting match, will depend on how you do, as it will have a direct impact on your everyday situations; people forget that the way they do things is according to how they feel.

Nobody teaches us about emotions, they are not taken seriously in schools as a necessary subject in the education of pupils. Today science helps to understand how emotions work, what they are for, how to regulate them and when they appear. We must consider that from 0 to 8 years old, beliefs are established, ways of thinking about what happens, science says that what happened to you in that age period has a lot of influence; it doesn't determine exactly how you will be as an adult, but it has a lot of influence.

Functions of the emotional system (finishes maturing at the age of four):

- Curiosity
- Excitement
- Attention
- Empatfa
- Memory

The prefrontal cortex is involved in what we consider most human:

- Ethics
- Moral
- Reasoning
- Social responsibility
- Emotional control
- Impulsivity
- Decision-making
- Planning for the future

The neural foundations:

- Excitement
- Curiosity
- Attention
- Awareness
- Mental processes
- Learning
- Memory and its consolidation
- I sound
- Biological rhythms

The system in charge of emotions is the hymbic system, which has a great influence not only on emotions, but also on memory because it is part of the hippocampus, which is the main memory centre of the brain. The hmbic system is made up of six structures:

- The thalamus, in charge of pleasure and pain
- am^gdala for nutrition, orality, protection and hostility
- The olfactory bulbs
- The septal region for sexuality

- The nucleus accumbens for desire
- The hippocampus for long-term memory

Motivation is important for learning anything. If we only strive to learn something, we release noradrenaline, the neurotransmitter of ene^a, but we will not release dopamine, which influences the desire to learn. Dopamine has not only been found to be the neurotransmitter responsible for pleasurable sensations, it is also involved in the coordination of muscle movements, in decision making and in the regulation of learning and memory. Without it we would not experience curiosity or motivation. According to the University College London Wellcome Trust Centre of Neuroimaging, dopamine affects decision-making, influencing the choice between one option and another.

Our dominant emotions are what determine how we live; this life is a complex mental process, with emotions acting as a trigger for each of our behaviours. However, you can learn to modify your emotional activations in response to stimuli, responding with new and better behaviours.

Emotions are a physiological resource that evolution has given us to adapt to certain environmental stimuli or to our thoughts in defence of survival, giving us the possibility to feel in a particular way and to act accordingly.

On the other hand, from a strictly biological point of view, emotions are previous neural learning circuits, they make the perceived information be recorded in a concrete way, improving the capacity to retain and learn; they are the glue of knowledge. Learning without emotions is learning that is difficult to retain, boring and demotivating. On a cerebral level, emotions activate attention, mental and cognitive processes, and also stimulate sensory and motor mechanisms. Emotions such as joy, love and surprise favour attentional states and are involved in learning, promoting long-term memory.

Neuroscientist Roger Sperry pointed out that mental states such as thoughts can act directly on the brain and can even affect the electrochemical activity of neurons. On the other hand, consciousness is the consequence of learning or experience.

So when we want an individual to learn, we not only need to create the means to stimulate positive emotions, but also to eliminate negative ones. Cultivate their self-esteem and you will be able to enhance their learning, a healthy self-esteem is fundamental for them to achieve optimal learning.

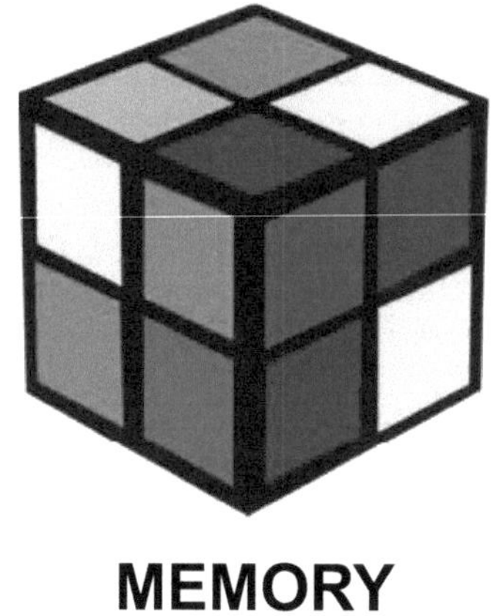

CHAPTER 5

MEMORY

MEMORY: FLEXIBLE AND ADAPTABLE

Memory begins to develop from birth, although it cannot be determined whether it is innate or not. However, recalling what we have learned whenever we want and making use of it in the context of a conversation or in an act of behaviour means making changes in the connections between neurons and morphological changes in the synapses as a result of learning and memory processes.

In 1900, the British Tim Bliss, Graham Collingridge and Richard Morris discovered the existence of synapses between neurons. They investigated that for the conformation of the memory something had to occur in the synapses, nevertheless, when they understood that we have approximately 100 thousand million neurons and each one achieves 5000 synapses, that is to say, about 500 billions of cerebral connections, they determined that the search would be interminable. On the other hand, in 1973 they observed that when applying an electrical stimulation they provoked a synapse in a cerebral zone now known as hippocampus, an essential area for the memory. This was when the term brain plasticity was first coined.

There are two types of memory: long-term memory and short-term memory. Long-term memory is the one that allows you to function every day, as well as regulating your vocabulary; short-term memory allows you to retain information.

There is also the so-called working memory. This is of limited capacity, so it is confused with short-term memory, but they are not the same: working memory retains information temporarily so that you can reason and make decisions, short-term memory only retains it. This means that, if you are one of the people who has a more developed working memory, you group information more deeply and remember more details about an experience, making you believe that you have already experienced it.

The brain is capable of anatomical and functional modification during the individual's lifetime, so that memory is flexible and adaptable. The latter makes learning possible.

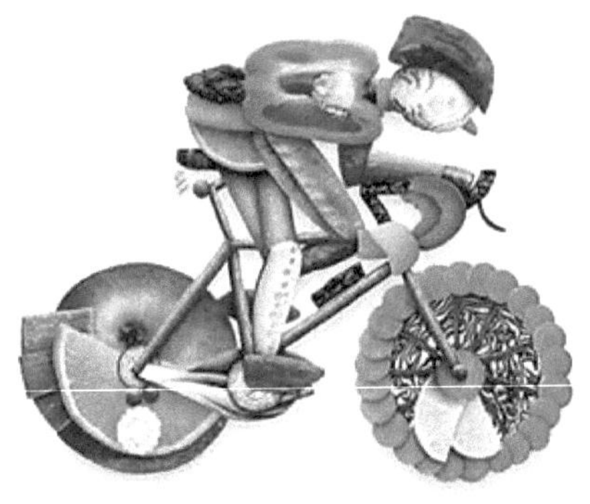

NUTRITION

NUTRITION: A LEARNING JUNCTURE

The brain is made up of neurons that communicate with each other by means of chemical substances known as

neurotransmitters. Learning, being one of our most complex functions, requires a level of attention - regulated by good muscular stimulation, as mentioned in chapter 2 - and an adequate state of alertness to be able to process the information received by our senses and use it when required; this is where nutrition plays a very important role.

Mexican nutritionist Mauricio Urtiaga explained to me at some point that we should consider the nutrients that are geared towards better concentration and memory stimulation. For his part, Garde warns that when it comes to nutrients, it is best to distribute them over five meals a day: the highest amounts should be at breakfast and lunch, leaving dinner at the lowest level but higher than lunch and afternoon snack.

According to several studies, poor nutrition and malnutrition in childhood affect behaviour and school performance as children grow up. Harvard University and Massachusetts General Hospital (USA) found that children with poor nutrition were prone to learning difficulties and attitude problems reflected in irritability, aggressiveness, difficulty understanding and lack of interest.

Similarly, it is necessary to mention junk food, as it affects learning for several reasons: by consuming it, the body receives empty calories, which are given to you in the form of

momentary feeling of satisfaction, but after a while you get hungry. Thus, your body does not have enough energy, which causes anxiety and lack of concentration, situations that will impede the cognitive process. In addition, when you consume too many calories, especially carbohydrates, you will feel sick to your stomach, dizziness, headache, tiredness and drowsiness, which will make it difficult for you to pay attention when learning.

Adequate nutrition should be a matter of public knowledge that should not be ignored. Its most damaging effects are not seen instantly but over time; if we were talking about sport, this would require other considerations for the proper performance of the athlete.

Here are some tables taken from the book *Feed Your Brain* by Ingrid Kiefer and Udo Zifko, for a proper nutrition.

FOR CONCENTRATION	
Carbohydrates	Cereals, fruits, vegetables.
L^quids	Aguamineral , infusions no sugary drinks.
Iron	Beef, pumpkin seeds, sesame, soy flour, oats, parsley, spinach, broccoli, lentils.
Chlorophyll	spinach, lettuce, peas, olives, herbs aromatic herbs, green plants.
Tryptophan	It is the precursor of serotonin which is related to good mood and learning. It is found in foods such as cheese and fish,
	rice, oat flakes.
Vitamin B1	It is involved in the metabolism of neurotransmitters. It is present in

	cereals whole grains, oats, sunflower seeds, pulses, nuts and pork.
Magnesium	Participate at the metabolism energetic. Present in cereals, pumpkin seeds , fruits dried.
Boron	Fruit, vegetables, nuts.

FOR MEMORY	
Phenylalanine	It is the precursor of noradrenaline, adrenaline and dopamine. Although some people are hypersensitive, it is needed to make dopamine, which is involved in the control of movement and wakefulness. It is important for memory. Found in soybeans, cheese, mam, almonds, wheat germ, tuna, beef, veal beef, trout and beetroot.
Serine, Methionine	Fish, chicken, soya, beef, nuts, broccoli, spinach, bread potatoes.
Vitamin B1	Whole grains, sunflower seeds, pulses, nuts, pork.
Lecithin (choline, phosphatidylcholine)	Precursor of acetylcholine. Found in egg yolk, soybeans, meat, meat, meat products, eggs and fish.
Cafe	Recent research confirms that caffeine improves long-term memory when taken after learning. While this beneficial effect of caffeine is already known, the substance has been given before the learning exercise, which has been shown to improve long-term memory. which made it difficult to separate the influence of caffeine on memory from its other effects, including an increase in alertness. However, the harmful effects in stressful situations have already been mentioned, and the fact that it does not increase our concentration, concentration and

	alertness has already been mentioned. concentration, but only a state of alertness.

FOR LEARNING CAPACITY	
Calcium	Necessary for the transmission of information between neurons. Found in milk and milk products, poppy seeds, figs, sesame, soya, nuts, whole grains, broccoli, wheat germ, oat flakes, green leafy vegetables, legumes and parsley.
Iodine	It is an important antioxidant. Found in iodised salt, sea fish, seaweed, spinach and eggs.
Carbohydrates	Supply glucosaparala ene^a production. It is found in cereals, fruits and vegetables.
Iron	Involved in the transport of
	oxygen. Present in red meat, pumpkin seeds, sesame, soy flour, millet, poppy seeds, parsley, spinach, yeast, watercress, peas, broccoli and lentils.
L^quids	More than 80% of the brain is water. Dehydration can seriously impair learning and simply increasing the amount of water we drink per day can improve concentration and memory (mineral water, unsweetened herbal teas, green tea).

FOR INFORMATION RETRIEVAL	
Tyrosine	Involved in the production of adrenaline and dopamine. Sources are beef, fish and dairy products.
Serine, methionine	Precursor of acetylcholine. Present in fish, chicken, soya, beef, nuts, broccoli, spinach, wholemeal bread and potatoes.

FOR THE TRANSMISSION OF INFORMATION	
Omega-3 fatty acids	It is the structural component of the membranes of the nervous system. It is found in fish.
Cinc	Component of enzymes. Its deficiency contributes to depression, violent

	behaviour, hyperactivity and and problems with
	learning. It is found in wheat germ, seeds of pumpkin, beef, eggs, milk, cheese, fish, carrots, wholemeal bread and potatoes.

PAR	IA ATTENTION
Tyrosine	Beef, fish, dairy products.

FOR INTELLECTUAL PERFORMANCE	
Carbohydrates	Cereals, fruits, vegetables.
Lysine	Milk and dairy products, egg, tuna, beef, pork, soya, wheat germ, lentils, chicken, manL
Asparagine	Asparagus.
Iron	Red meat, pumpkin seeds, sesame, soy flour, oats, parsley, spinach, broccoli, lentils.
L^quids	Watermineral , infusions, no sugary drinks.

OTHER NUTRIENTS FOR OVERALL BRAIN HEALTH	
Copper	Fish, cereals, nuts, chocolate, cocoa, green tea, coffee, green vegetables.
Phosphorus	Sausages, beef, cheese, dried fruit and nuts, pulses, fruit, vegetables.
Flavonoids	They help the communication between neurons (synapses), reduce neuronal ageing and improve
	memory, you can find them in dark chocolate, red wine, grapes, berries, citrus fruits, citrus fruits, celery, apples, onions, cabbage, tomatoes, aubergines, soya beans and cocoa. Phenolic acids (lettuce, potatoes, nuts, green and black tea).
Phytoestrogens	Legumes, cereals cereals, vegetable oils, pulses.
Sulphur	Onion, leek, garlic.
Frtic acid	Cereals cereals, oils vegetables, pulses.
Folic acid	Spinach, lettuce, asparagus,

	cereals, tomato, cucumber, Liver.
Vitamin B6	Chicken, pork, fish, vegetables, potatoes, whole grains.
Vitamin B12	Beef, eggs, milk, fish, fish, fish products.
Quercetin, curcuma, sodium	Onion, curcuma at powder, olives, parmesan cheese, pate.
Alpha lipoic acid	A powerful regulator of cellular balance, it helps to combat stress and neutralise free radicals. It is found in vegetables such as kidney, heart and liver, as well as in green vegetables such as spinach and broccoli.
Vitamin E	Improves neuronal activity and prevents oxidation membranes neuronal membranes. found in curry, asparagus, walnuts, mam, olives and olive oil.
L-glutamine	For produce acidogamma-aminobufric acid (GABA) in the brain. It is found in pork and
	cow as well as sunflower seeds.

FOR EVERY MOMENT IN PROPER NUTRITION

To prevent afternoon slump: light, protein-rich food.

To study well: foods rich in carbohydrates.

Breakfast: to start the day with energy, the first thing to do is to get the right amount of fuel. Carbohydrates (cereals and fruit) will be the main thing, then a small amount of protein for the synthesis of neurotransmitters, attention and a positive attitude. Cereals have vitamin B1, ideal for good concentration.

The test day: light, high-protein foods.

A mid-morning snack to maintain concentration: a piece of fruit and a low-fat dairy product can prevent us from being too hungry at midday. Be careful, because if we have not had a good breakfast, instead of a snack we may need carbohydrates and proteins, so a sandwich with cheese and chicken will be ideal to achieve a good level of concentration.

CONCLUSION

Conscious as a professional of physical activity and passionate about the world of neurosciences, which every day bring new discoveries, I am encouraged to take this step - perhaps daring - to offer a proposal of pedagogical intervention from the court and the classroom, because it will be very difficult for a neuroscientist to give us a course that provides us with information about motor action. After having written this book, I can tell you that learning something new means changing your brain, hence the importance of knowing the different brain functions in relation to learning, from the processing of the information you receive thanks to your senses, to the sensory processing and the execution of motor acts, where elements such as attention, memory and emotion, as well as adequate nutrition, play a relevant role in improving the teaching-learning process.

It is clear to me that there is still a lot to know and I know that the writing you have in your hands is only an attempt to make known a proposal that involves attentional processes that help in our daily work as educators and trainers, with the purpose of having an impact on the quality of our teaching. I would have liked to give you more information, as well as more practical resources, but my intention is not to give you a recipe, but a vision of what you can achieve when you better understand the application of the attentional process that involves these four elements.

I invite you to try this new binomial, which combines physical activity and the brain to offer transcendent learning to those you teach. (Ratey, 2008), said: "If exercise could be prescribed in the form of a pill, it would be the medicine of the century", the challenge is that you know the right time and type of activity, depending on the context, age and interests of those to whom you direct it. Now, after having done the present, we will be able to talk in the near future about designing neuromotor programmes for cognitive and/or motor sport learning at different ages.

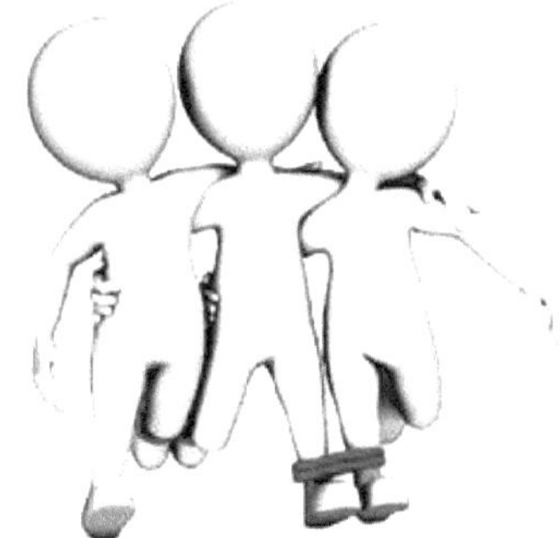

■ Attention

■ Sensoperception

□ Memory

■ Excitement

Sitting in a circle, each player will have a tennis ball which he will pass to his partner on the right, rolling it with his hand without turning to look at it. At the same time they will look to their left side to receive the ball from their partner with their left hand, repeating the same action. The intention is that the balls are rolling at the same time without anyone making a mistake. Then they can do it to the other side.

- **Variants**: bouncing the ball between two players, throwing the ball

through the air, passing it under the legs, etc. The balls can be of different sizes, textures and weights.

- **Material:** Tennis balls.
- **Aspects to consider:** Explain that they must calculate the force and speed with which they will throw the ball, they can do this by talking to organise themselves and then no one can talk.

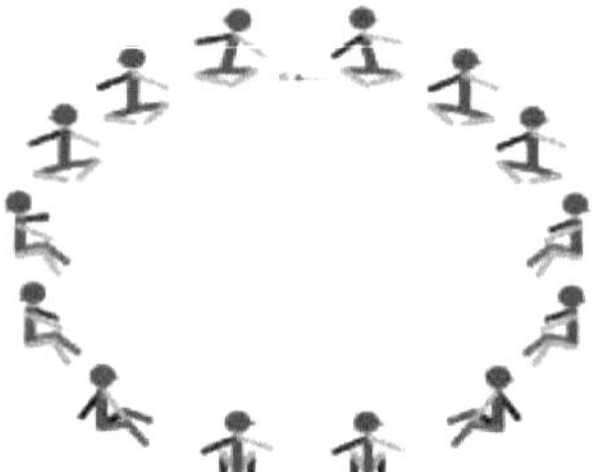

Standing in a circle, each player has a tennis ball which he passes to his partner on the right, bouncing it with his right hand without turning to look at him. At the same time he/she will look to his/her left side to receive the ball from the partner with the left hand, repeating the same action. The intention is that the balls are bouncing at the same time without anyone making a mistake. They can then bounce to the other side.

- **Variants**: Throwing it up in the air to your partner without

over the height of your face, do it at different speeds, etc. Balls can be of different sizes, textures and weights.

- **Material:** Tennis balls. Balls can be of different materials, sizes, textures and weights.
- **Aspects to consider:** Explain that they must calculate the force and speed with which they will throw the ball, they can do this by talking to organise themselves and then no one can talk.

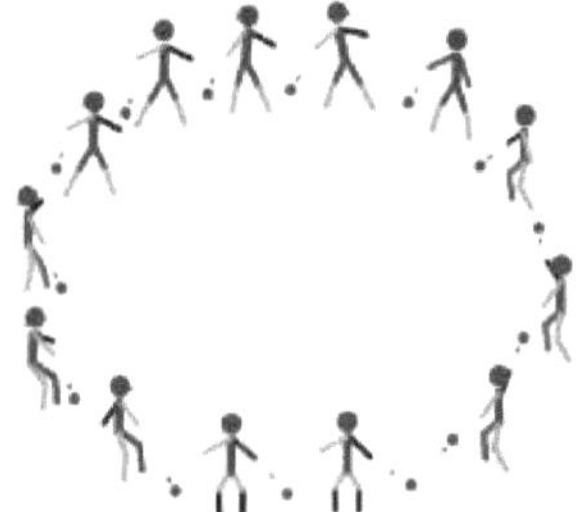

Standing in a circle, each player will have a tennis ball that will bounce so that it bounces up to the height of their face; at the same time they will take a lateral step to the right trying to catch the ball that their partner bounced and they will repeat the action, then they can do it to the other side. The intention is to make sure that nobody misses the ball and that they all manage to do it at the same pace.

- **Variants**: Throwing it upwards; throwing it, clapping your hands and catching your partner's ball, etc. Balls can be of different sizes, textures and weights.
- **Material:** Tennis balls. Balls can be of different materials, sizes, textures and weights.
- **Aspects to consider:** Explain that they must calculate the force and speed with which they will

throw the ball, they can do this by talking to organise themselves and then no one can talk.

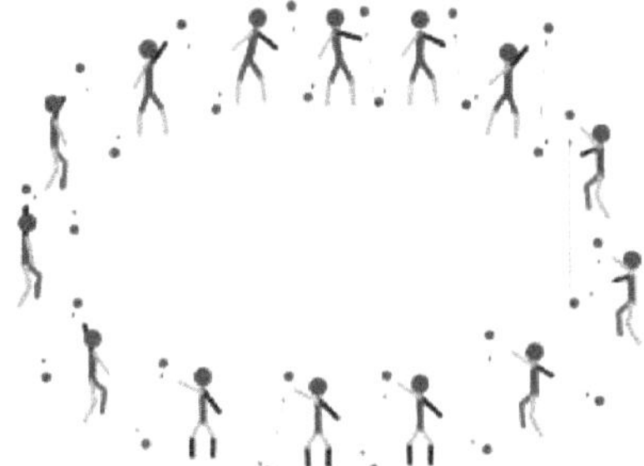

In pairs and standing up, each player will have a ball and each will hold it in their right hand, at the signal they will throw it to their partner who will catch it with their left hand and at the same time change hands to repeat the action. The intention is that they manage to keep a rhythm in their throws and do not drop the ball.

- **Variants**: Throwing with the left hand, doing the same while walking, etc.
- **Material**: tennis balls. Balls can be of different materials, sizes, textures and weights.
- **Aspects to consider**: Explain that they must calculate the force and speed with which they will throw the ball, they can do this by talking to organise themselves and then no one can talk.

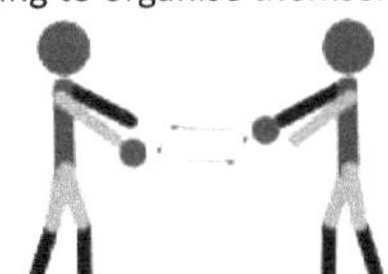

In pairs and standing up, each player will have a ball and hold it in their right hand, at the signal one will throw the ball to their partner from above and the other will throw it so that it bounces between them. Both will catch the ball with their left hand and when they receive it they will pass it to their right hand to repeat the action. The intention is that they manage to keep a rhythm in their throws and do not drop the ball.

- **Variants**: Throwing with the left hand, doing the same while walking, etc.
- **Material**: tennis balls. Balls can be of different materials, sizes, textures and weights.
- **Aspects to consider**: Explain that they must calculate the force and speed with which they will throw the ball, they can do this by talking to organise themselves and then no one will be able to talk.

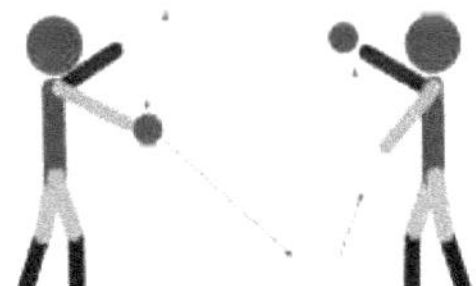

In pairs, seated or kneeling, you will have a ball each; each one will have it in the right hand and at the signal both will throw it rolling to the partner so that the balls arrive at the same time, both will catch it with the left hand and when they receive it they will pass it to the right hand to repeat the action. The intention is that they manage to keep a rhythm in their throws and do not drop the ball.

- **Variants**: Throw with the left hand, do the
same at different speeds, bouncing it, throwing it in the air, etc.
- **Material**: tennis balls. Balls can be of different materials, sizes, textures and weights.
- **Aspects to consider**: Explain that they must calculate the force and speed with which they will throw the ball, they can do this by talking to organise themselves and then no one will be able to talk.

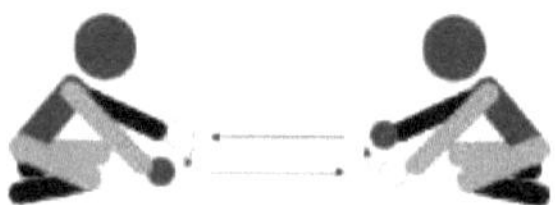

Individually each person will have their own ball which they must throw as high as possible with their right hand, while the ball is in the air they will sit down to catch it. The intention is not to drop the ball.

- **Variations**: Throw with the left hand, do the same by bouncing it, etc. etc. etc.
- **Material:** tennis balls. Balls can be of different materials, sizes, textures and weights.
- **Aspects to consider:** Explain that they should calculate the force and speed with which they will throw the ball.

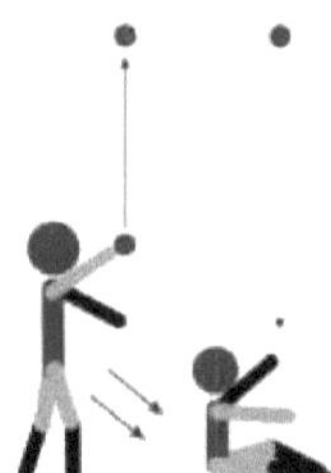

Sitting in a circle, a partner will be chosen who will be the one to guess who Morpheus is, he/she will turn his/her back to his/her partners so that they can decide who Morpheus is and will fall asleep in a chair previously agreed by the group. The intention of the activity is that whoever is standing up will try to guess who Morpheus is and be attentive to the group at all times to find out. When they find out, they will change roles.

- **Variants**: Using coloured flags to give the signal.
- Material: Free.
- **Points to consider:** Explain to the group that everyone should be completely silent.

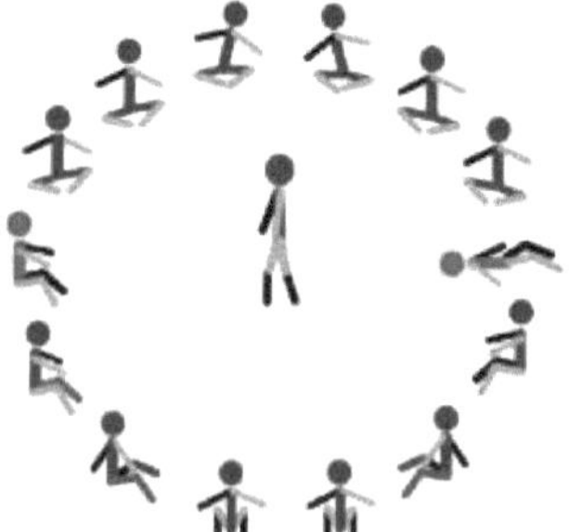

In a designated area, hoops will be distributed forming a large circle, in the centre of which there will be one person and inside each hoop there will be the rest of the group, no more than one person per hoop. At the signal, everyone must run to a hoop that is not theirs and not the one next to them; the one in the centre without a hoop will try to get to one, the one without a hoop will go to the centre and the same action will be repeated. The intention is that at all times they should be attentive so as not to run out of hoops.

- **Variants**: In pairs holding hands, threes, etc.
- Material: Hoops.
- **Aspects to consider:** Explain to the group that they should not go to the hoops next to them and be careful not to collide.

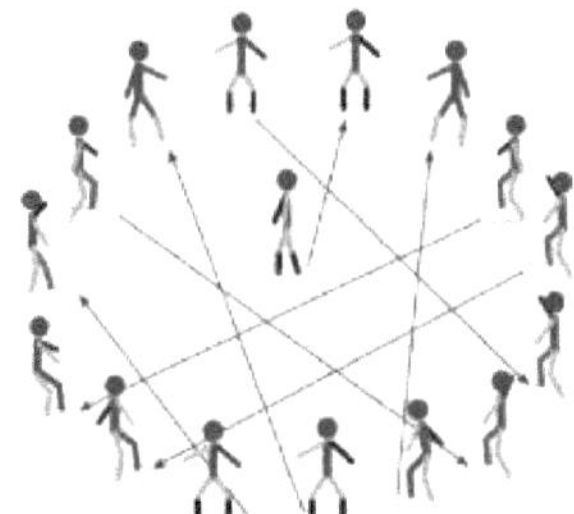

Forming a large circle with a football, someone will stand in the middle of the circle, at the signal they will start to pass to each other and the one in the middle will try to take the ball away from them, each time they manage to pass the ball, everyone will count the number of passes they have made out loud. When the student in the middle manages to take the ball away, he/she will take the place of the person who took the ball away and start again.

- **Variants**: Throw a ball in the air, make it two at a time.

centre.

- **Material:** Football or plastic ball.
- **Things to consider:** Balls can be of different materials and sizes.

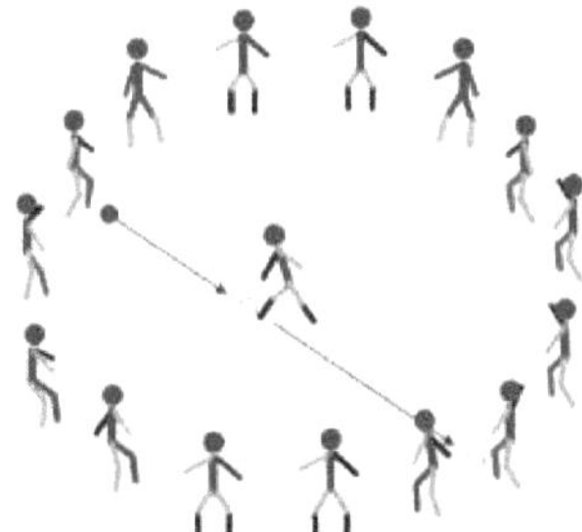

In pairs and distributed in an area, one of them will stand with a ball in each hand and his arms stretched out to the sides, his partner will stand at a distance of four metres and with his back to his partner. At the signal he/she must turn and try to catch the ball that his/her partner has dropped without it bouncing more than once. The intention is for him to be attentive to who will catch the ball at the signal.

- **Variants**. Throwing the ball in the air, bouncing the ball hard.
- **Material:** Tennis ball or sponge.
- **Things to consider:** Balls can be of different materials and sizes.

In pairs and distributed in an area, one will stand with a ball in each hand and arms stretched out to the sides, his partner will stand at a distance of four metres and with his back to his partner. At the signal whoever is taking the balls will shout right or left and the one who has his back turned must turn and try to catch the ball that his partner said without the ball bouncing more than once. The intention is to be attentive to who catches the ball at the signal.

- **Variants**: Throwing the ball in the air, bouncing the ball hard.
- **Material:** Tennis ball or sponge.

- **Things to consider:** Balls can be of different materials and sizes.

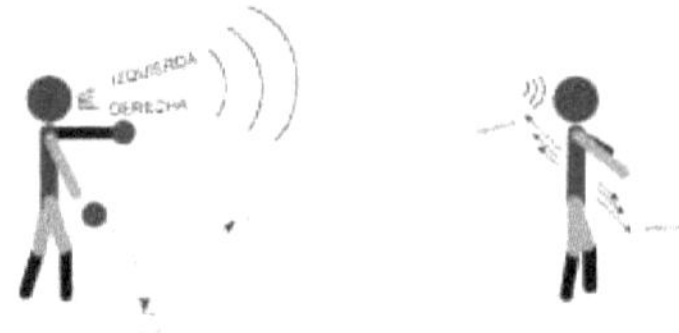

In pairs and distributed in an area, one will stand with a ball in each hand and arms stretched out to the sides, his partner will stand at a distance of four metres and with his back to his partner, at the signal whoever is taking the balls will mention an air animal and will drop the right ball, if he says a land animal he will drop the left ball and the one with his back must turn and try to catch the ball that his partner indicated according to the animal mentioned, the ball must not give more than one bounce. The intention is to be attentive to who will catch the ball at the signal.

- **Variants:** Throwing the ball in the air, bouncing the ball hard, bouncing it ball.
- **Material:** Tennis ball or sponge.
- **Things to consider:** Balls can be of different materials and sizes.

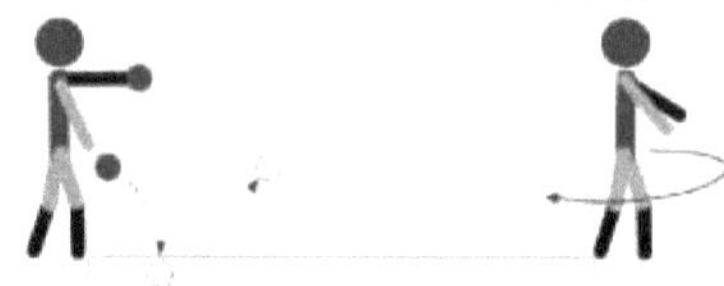

There will be hoops in front of two teams facing each other, at the signal a member of team one will run to put a panuelo inside a hoop and immediately one of team 2 will come out to do the same, the objective is to form a cat with the panuelos and prevent the other team from doing so.

- **Variants:** Do it with objects that are difficult to transport, using blindfolds and your team gwa.
- **Material:** Hoops, bandanas or bandanas.
- **Aspects to consider:** Must come out one by one from each team

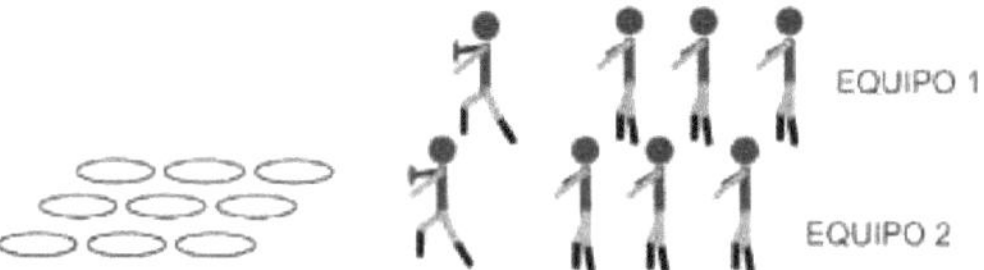

With hoops on the floor, two teams will try to make a cat by putting up sticks but when they leave the cat they must drive a basketball.

- **Variants:** These can be different types of balls, bouncing them or throwing them.
- **Material:** Various balls.
- **Points to consider:** Each player must wait his or her turn.

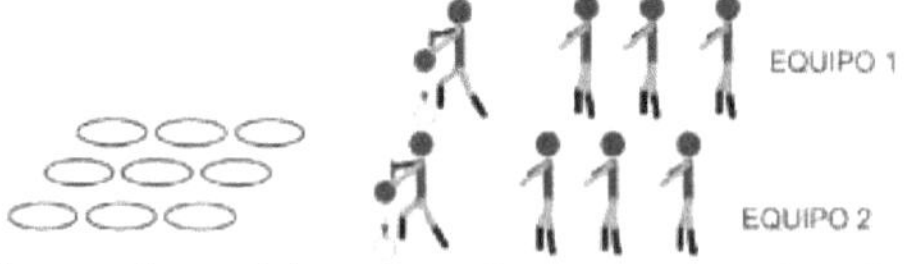

Placed in pairs, one will try to clap and the other will try to prevent the other from clapping, at the signal they change roles.

- **Variants:** One place, running, all against all.
- **Material:** None
- **Aspects to consider:** The indication will only be to prevent the partner from clapping, creativity

comes into play, they can clap with feet, knees, etc.

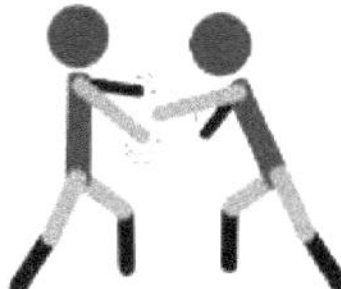

In pairs, one blindfolded person will try to hit a balloon with their head to avoid it falling to the ground, their partner will guide them and show them where to move in order to achieve the objective and at the same time make sure they don't crash. At the signal they will change places.

- **Variants**: Using two balloons, bouncing a ball, etc.
- **Material:** Balloon and bandana.
- **Aspects to consider:** Take care that the working area is sufficient so as not to collide with colleagues.

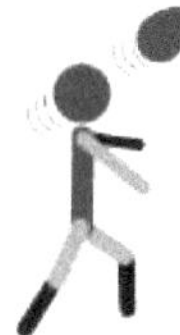

Hoops are placed on the floor and on a sheet of paper they will draw them, marking some of them with "x" representing mines. A blindfolded player will walk between the hoops and his teammates will guide him, but when he steps on a hoop marked with an "x" on the drawing, everyone will shout "boom" and another player will try not to step on it.

- **Variants**: Passing in pairs, trios, etc.
- **Material:** Hoops and bandanas.
- **Aspects to consider:** Fix the hoops with maskin or paint them to avoid accidents when stepping on them.

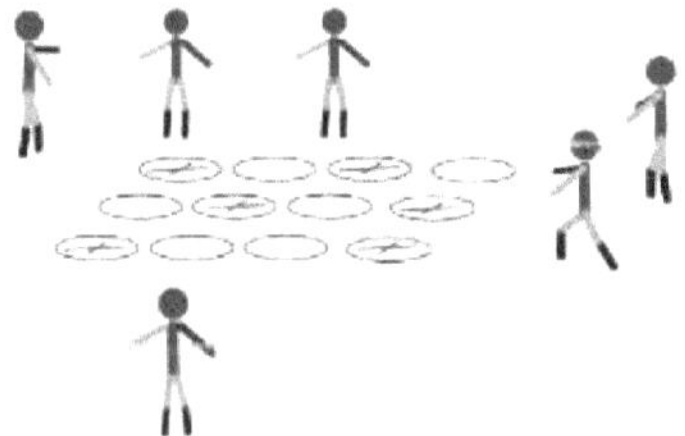

Playing in pairs, they play rock, paper, scissors and the winner must turn and run to a set mark, if he/she reaches the mark without being touched, he/she will get a point. The action is repeated until 10 points are scored.

- **Variants**: Running while manipulating a ball.
- **Material:** None or balls.
- **Aspects to consider:** In order to be caught it must be touched in back.

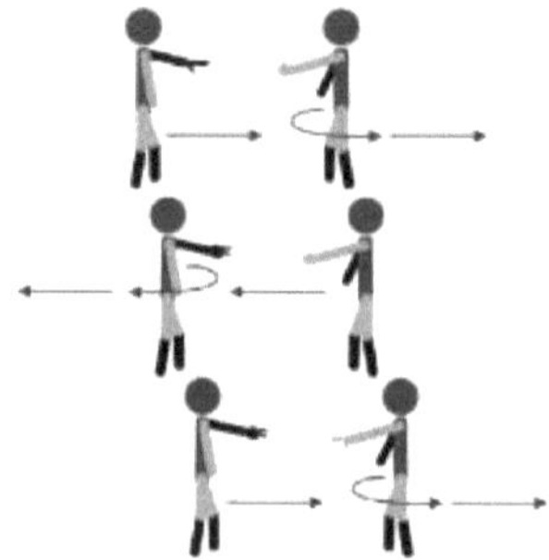

Two players will lead a rope to all sides holding it with their hands and lifting it as high as possible, two teams will play volleyball but the rope will be mobile and if they are touched by it they will lose a point.

- **Variants**: Play with different sizes of balls.
- **Material:** Balls and a long rope.
- **Points to consider:** Points will be cumulative but each time the ball is dropped or touched by the rope, one point will be subtracted.

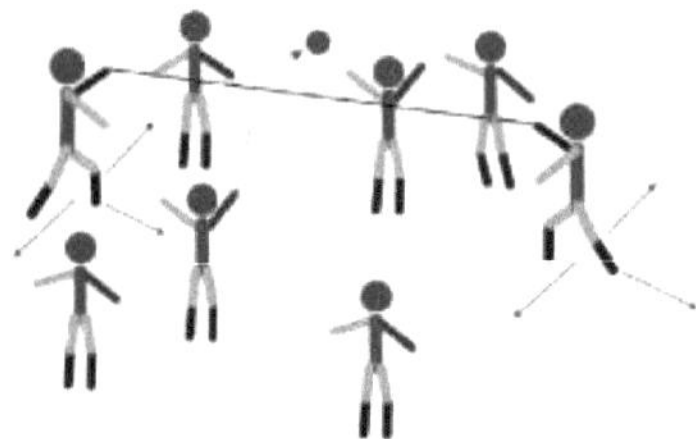

The players will be divided into two teams, the members of one team will do different poses and the other team will have 5 seconds to memorise them, then they will try to do exactly the same poses. They can use a photo with their mobile phone to check if they succeeded or not.

- **Variants**: Imitating animals, sport poses, etc.
- **Material:** none.
- **Aspects to consider:** Time to remember poses is determined by the team.

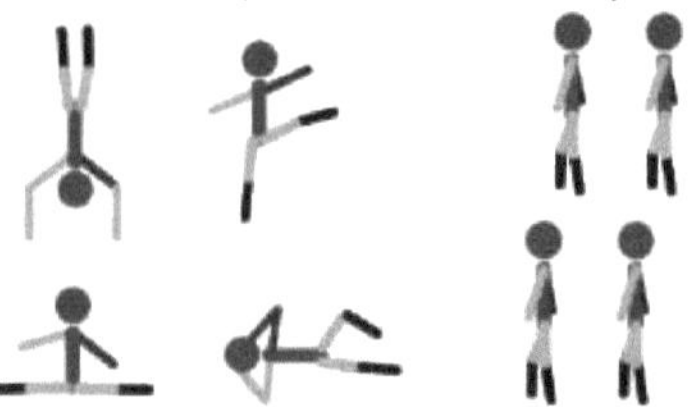

In pairs, one will be blindfolded, the other will perform a position for his partner to try to guess it by touch and when he thinks he knows what it looks like he will perform it, he will have three attempts.

- **Variants**: Animal poses, sports, etc.
- **Material:** Bandanas.
- **Aspects to consider:** The time to achieve replicate the pose will be determined by the players.

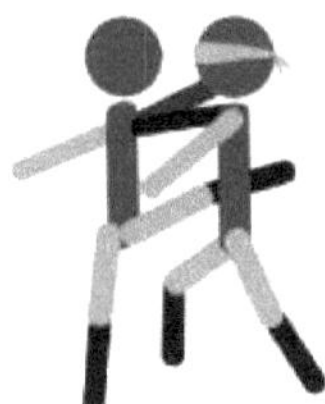

Two players will hold a rope, one blindfolded player will jump continuously at different heights, the other player will indicate when and at what height to jump.

- **Variants**: Use different materials on the rope.
- **Material:** ropes.
- **Aspects to consider:** Determine spaces that are not dangerous in case of falls when jumping. Mats can be placed.

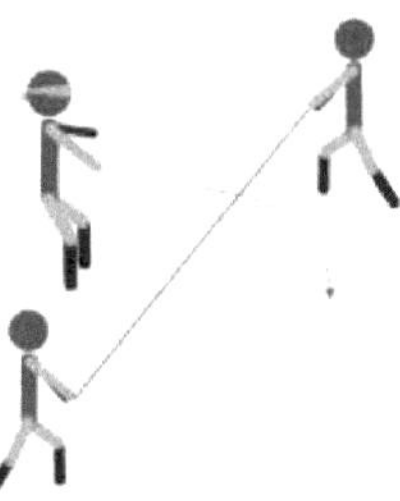

GLOSSARY

Amygdala Almond-shaped brain structure composed of a set of nuclei with different histological characteristics. It is located within the temporal lobe. It is part of the circuits involved in the elaboration of emotion and motivation and in the control of the autonomic or vegetative nervous system.

Learning A process that an organism goes through with experience and by which behaviour is modified. It is closely associated with memory processes. It involves plastic changes in the brain that are now believed to be related to synaptic activity.

Visual areas of the cerebral cortex Based on functional and connection studies, the visual areas of the cerebral cortex have been subdivided into more than 25 different areas. The main ones include: V1 = Primary striate visual area. V2 = Visual area situated around V1 from which it receives information; V3 = Visual area that receives information from V2 and projects to V4 and V5; V4 = Visual area situated between the borders of the temporal, occipital and parietal cortex; V5 or MT (medial temporal) = Visual area situated in the medial temporal cortex; MST (medial superior temporal) = Visual area situated in the medial and superior temporal lobule.

Attention Neuropsychological process that is able to select among several stimuli the one to which it responds. Several types of attention with different neural substrates are known today.

Cerebellum This is an organ situated posterior to the bulb and the pons. It contains the intermediate part or vermis and the two cerebral hemispheres. It consists of a cerebellar cortex and deep nuclei. It plays an important role in the control of voluntary motor activity and in the processes of learning and memory.

Brain At present it is a term that is not clearly defined and agreed upon. In general it refers to that part of the central nervous system (CNS) which is contained within the cranial cavity, excluding the brainstem and cerebellum.

Neural circuit A series of neural connections in which signal transmission is accomplished by the action and interaction of various neurotransmitters and which code for specific functions.

Code A series of symbols or rules used with specific meaning that make up a communication system.

Neural communication The process of communication and transmission of information between neurons using a particular code.

Cerebral cortex Neuronal layer of the outer surface of the brain in humans and higher organisms. In humans, its total surface area is about 2,200 cm^2 and its thickness ranges from 1.3 to 4.5 mm, with a volume of 600 cm^3 . Typically, there are six distinct layers, which exist in more than 90 percent of the total cortex.

Cingulate cortex The medial part of the cerebral cortex which is part of the Kmbic system and is related to the
brain mechanisms involved in the processes of attention, emotion and motivation.

Frontal cortex Refers to the entire cortex of the frontal lobe, which includes the anterior pole of the cerebral hemispheres from the Rolando fissure.

Parietal cortex Cortex related to somatic sensation, language and visuospatial processing and control.

Prefrontal cortex Association cortex located in the most rostral part of the frontal lobe. Its neurophysiological definition and limits are given by projections from the dorsomedial nucleus of the thalamus. It is subdivided into several other areas: orbital and dorsal prefrontal cortex (in the primate) or dorsal medial and orbital (in the rat). Among the many functions in which it is involved are the control of the emotional world through the Kmbic system, working memory, programming or planning of voluntary motor actions and actions to be performed in the immediate future, and inhibitory function of both external and internal influences.

Premotor cortex Area of the cerebral cortex located rostral or anterior to the primary motor area with which it is intimately connected. It is thought to be involved in the cortical programming of voluntary movements.

Temporal cortex Part of the neocortex involved in processing auditory and visual information, emotions and declarative memory.

Visual cortex Part of the cerebral cortex located in the occipital pole and related to vision.

Corpus callosum Commissure between the two cerebral hemispheres. A band of nerve fibres that runs from one side of the brain to the other and connects the cerebral hemispheres, integrating their functions and allowing the neurons of the two hemispheres to synchronise their activity.

Emotion Behavioural and subjective reaction produced by information from the external or internal world (memory) of the individual. It is accompanied by neurovegetative phenomena. The Kmbic system is an important part of the brain involved in the processing of emotional behaviour.

Basal ganglia Series of nuclei located at the base of the cerebral hemispheres (hence the name). Called ganglia after the term applied by 19th century histologists to large groups of neurons. They are made up of the caudate and putamen nuclei (both of which are called the striatum) and the globus pallidus with its outer and inner segments. Functionally, the striatum-pallidum complex acts in connection with the subthalamic nucleus (networked with the pallidum) and the substantia nigra (pars compacta and pars reticularis, interconnected with the striatum). The basal ganglia receive information from large areas of the cerebral cortex and the hymbic system. Their function is related to motor planning and motor memory.

Cerebral hemisphere Each of the two large anterodorsal lobes of the telencephalon of the vertebrate brain.

Hippocampus Circumvolution located in the anteromedial region of the temporal lobe, resulting from the internalisation, in mammals, of an archaic cortex developed in reptiles and primitive mammals. It consists mainly of two structures: the gyrus or dentate fascia and Ammon's horn. It consists of three layers (molecular, granular and polymorphic). It is part of the Kmbic system. Fundamental structure in the recording of different types of memories.

Hypothalamus A structure located below the thalamus and above the optic chiasm and sella turcica that is involved in the regulation of the neurovegetative and endocrine systems. It forms a fundamental part of the neural control circuits for food intake, water, sexuality and temperature. It is made up of neuronal clusters or nuclei.

Lobule Subdivision of an organ or part of an organ delimited by its shape, fissures, grooves, septa, etc. In the brain, the lobule is each of the parts of the cerebral cortex separated by fissures.

Frontal lobe One of the four main divisions of the cerebral cortex. It is located anterior to the central fissure or Roland's fissure. It is involved in the programming and execution of motor acts, including speech, and in the control of emotional behaviour.

hmbic lobule Gyrus and associated structures with the medial and basal surface of the cerebral hemisphere surrounding the superior brain stem, cingulate gyrus, isthmus, hippocampus, parahippocampal gyrus and uncus, and amygdala. It plays an important role in behaviour and emotion.

Occipital lobule One of the four main divisions of the cerebral cortex. It forms the posteriormost part of the cerebral hemispheres. Its rostral hemisphere is located at the parietooccipital fissure. It is primarily and principally concerned with the processing of visual information.

Parietal lobule One of the four main divisions of the cerebral cortex. It is bounded on its anterior border by the fissure of Rolando (external face) and by the internal perpendicular fissure or parietooccipital sulcus (internal face). Distinctions are made between the ascending parietal gyrus (postcentral), the superior parietal gyrus and the inferior parietal gyrus.

Temporal lobe One of the four divisions of the cerebral cortex. It is situated ventral to the Sylvian fissure, on the outer surface of which are the superior, middle and inferior convolutions.

Memory Ability to recall previously learned responses.

Memory, consolidation Process by which memory short term memory is converted into long term memory.

Short-term memory Memory that temporarily retains information (minutes-hours). Type of memory prior to its transformation into long-term memory. Information of this type is immediately accessible to consciousness.

Long-term memory Long-term memory, in some cases for life.

Active or working memory A concept originally proposed by Baddeley and Hitch that refers to a type of memory whose information is retained while it is being processed. It is now thought to be a collection of temporal capacities associated with different modalities. This type of memory is affected by lesion of the dorsolateral part of the prefrontal cortex.

Associative, declarative or explicit memory Ability to remember an event in which the variables of space (location of the event), time (variable time elapsed since the event) and symbolic aspect of the event (a certain event and not another with certain characteristics) have been associated. Hippocampal lesions produce deficits in these characteristics.

Procedural or implicit memory Type of sensorimotor memory that involves habits, behaviours and skills such as, for example, riding a bicycle, playing golf or playing the piano.

Neuroscience The discipline that studies the development, structure, function, pharmacology and pathology of the nervous system.

Neuroeducation refers to the application of knowledge about how the brain works integrated with psychology, sociology and medicine in an attempt to improve and enhance both the learning and memory processes of students and better teaching in teachers. Neuroeducation includes helping to detect psychological or brain processes that may interfere with learning and memory and with education.

Feeling Conscious perception of emotions. They are the specifically human addition to emotions.

Synapse Term coined by Charles Sherrington to mean the junction or contact between two neurons. They can be both electrical and chemical. Three parts of the synapse are to be considered: the presynapse, the synaptic space and the postsynapse. At the qwmical synapse, the interneuronal signal is transmitted by a qwmical substance released from the presynaptic terminal. This interacts with specific receptors located at the postsynaptic terminal. The number of synapses of each neuron is highly variable, but is usually large, approximately one mammalian motor neuron has about 5,000 synapses. A single Purkinje cell in the cerebral cortex has about 90,000 synapses.

Hobic system Generic concept with imprecise anatomical and functional delimitations. It refers to the set of brain areas that are supposed to form circuits that encode the personal world of emotion (pleasure, anger, aggression, etc.) and motivation (food and water intake, sexual activity, etc.). These include: cingulate gyrus, parahippocampal gyrus, hippocampus, am^gdala, septum, nucleus accumbens, hypothalamus and orbitofrontal cortex.

Active rhythmic process, usually recurrent with a 24-hour cycle.

Sleep, stages Each sleep cycle goes through five stages depending on the type of brain activity represented by the electroencephalogram. During stages 1 to 14 there is a progressive decrease in brain wave activity from an alpha rhythm to a delta rhythm. Stages 1 and 2 take up 50 percent of the time, and stages 3 and 4 take up 25 percent of the time. The fifth stage is paradoxical or REM sleep and occupies the remaining 25 per cent.

BIBLIOGRAPHICAL REFERENCES

Ansermet,F., Magistretti, P. A cada cual su cerebro. Buenos Aires: Katz Editores. 2006.

Bachrach E. (2015): Encambio: Learn how to change your brain to change your life and feel better. Conecta. Buenos Aires.

Blakemore, Sarah, Frith, U. How the brain learns. Buenos Aires: Ariel, 2005.

Cattaneo, L., & Rizzolatti, G. (2009). The mirror neuron system. Archives of Neurology

Cebolla, A. Garcia Campayo J. and Demarzo, M. (2014) Mindfulness and science. Madrid Alianza.

Chadodock, L., Erickson, K.I., Prakash, R.S., Kim, J.S., Voss,M.W., et al. (2010). A neuroimaging investigation of the association between aerobic fitness, hippocampal volume, and memory performance in preadolescent children. Brain Res 1358: 172183.

Collard P. (2014) The Little book of mindfulness. Journal of school health.

Fisher,K.W. (2007): Why mind, brain and education. 1-2.

Goleman, Daniel. Emociones destructivas. Buenos Aires: Ediciones B, 2003.

Kiefer, Ingrid, Zikko, Udo. Feed your brain. Buenos Aires: Obelisco, 2011.

Logatt G. C. (2015) Neuropsychoeducation for all. Argentina.

Monti et al. (2012). Aerobic Fiteness Enhances Relational Memory in Preadolescent Children: The Fit Kids Randomized ControlTrial .   [en   lmea][disonible at
http://www.sde.idaho.gov/site/csh/docs/
Hippocampus%20V22%289%29%202012Monti%20%283%29.pd f][Accessed: 28 September 2018].

Mora F. (2017): (cuando el cerebro juega con las ideas) Madrid. Alianza Editorial.

Punset, Eduardo, Mora, F., Bisquerra, R. Como educar las emociones. Esplugues de Llobregat: Edicion Faros Sant Joan De Deu, 2012.

Ratey, J. (2003). El cerebro: manual de instrucciones. Barcelona: Debolsillo.

Reyes C. (2018) The importance of concentration and focus of attention in sport. [En Knea] [Available at   :https://psicologiaymente.com/deporte/concentracion-
focus-attention-sport [Accessed: 09 September 2018].

Scholz, J., Klein, M. Learning transforms the brain. Mind and Brain Notebooks No. 4. 2013.

Ratey, J. (2008). Spark: The revolutionarynew science of excersice and the brain. New York: Little, Brown and Company.

Rosler, R. (2014) Cerebro y ejercicio aliados en el aprendizaje. Asociacion educar.

Rodriguez, N. (2016) Neuroeducacion para padres. Penguin Random House Grupo Editorial Espana.

Sousa D.A. (2014) Educational neuroscience. Mind, brain and education. Madrid: Narcea.

Suzuky, W. (2011). Excersice and Brian. [en Hnea][Available at
http://www.youtube.com/watch?v=LdDnPYr6R0o][Accessed: 12 August 2018].

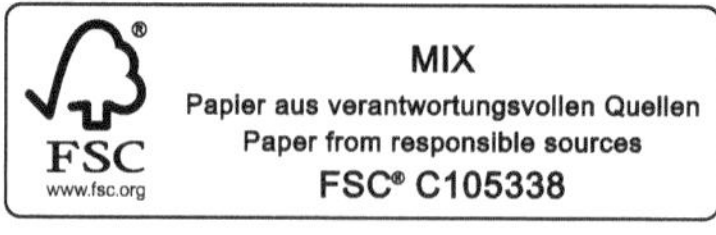

Printed by Books on Demand GmbH, Norderstedt / Germany